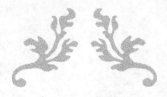

THE AUTOIMMUNE PALEO COOKBOOK

Lean and green wholesome paleolithic recipes for weekly meal plans

JESSICA COLLINS

this book has been derived from various sources. Please consult a licensed professional before attempting any techniques outlined in this book.

By reading this document, the reader agrees that under no circumstances is the author responsible for any losses, direct or indirect, which are incurred as a result of the use of information contained within this document, including, but not limited to, errors, omissions, or inaccuracies.

Table of Contents

INTRODUCTION

The paleo diet is eating that is concentrating on foods that our caveman ancestors would have eaten. It is a relatively simple diet, but it does require quite a bit of work. You need to eat unprocessed foods, limit your salt intake, eat healthy fats, and eat some fruit.

It allows you to avoid foods that have been associated with the disease. It helps reduce food cravings as it doesn't contain processed food full of sugar, fat, and carbs. It helps you to make better decisions as you can be more in tune with your body's needs. It is a low-carb, high protein diet, so it aids in weight loss and muscle gain. It is high in fat, so it suppresses hunger while providing energy for your body.

The paleo diet has several benefits for you. It is a very healthy diet that can help improve your body's overall health because you are not eating processed foods. Your diet will also help you look better and feel better as it removes junk food from your system.

Using the paleo diet cookbook can help you stick to the diet for the long term. All recipes are made with easy ingredients that focus on whole foods as opposed to processed products. As a bonus, all recipes are gluten-free! The paleo diet is appraised by many to be a healthy and balanced eating plan. This diet is based on the reliance that our body was meant to eat foods naturally. It primarily focuses on whole foods like fruits, vegetables, nuts, and seeds rather than processed foods to supply all of the necessary vitamins, minerals, and other nutrients to maintain and improve your health.

The paleo diet has been obtaining popularity over the last few years, especially among those interested in losing weight and enhance their overall health. Many people believe that this eating plan helps achieve both of those goals. The paleo diet cookbook is designed for beginners who are new to this eating plan.

The paleo diet encourages consuming whole foods with minimal processing or cooking. You can enjoy foods like meats, kinds of seafood, eggs, fruits, vegetables, and nuts without the addition of oils or other unhealthy additives. The paleo diet adopts high-fiber consumption and plenty of fruits and vegetables to help you stay healthy and fit. The paleo diet is a program that focuses on eating like it did in the Paleolithic Era. The paleo diet's mantra is that humans have an innate tendency to eat like our hunter-gatherer ancestors.

The paleo diet is constructed on the idea that modern man has become out-of-sync with his physiology. This out-of-sync can be attributed to the introduction of agriculture in the Neolithic era, which displaced our ancient hunter-gatherer ancestors. The theory goes that modern man is no longer fulfilling his physical requirements for food.

---

1. Chinese Steamed Eggs

Preparation time: 5 minutes

Cooking time: 15 minutes

Servings: 2

Ingredients:

- 2 eggs

- 1 cup of water

- Salt

- 1 Tbsp. of minced green onion

- 1 tsp. of sesame seeds

Directions:

1. Beat the eggs with a fork, add water and salt.

2. Filter the compound into two heat resistant bowls.

3. Boil some water into a pan, when the water starts boiling put the bowl into a bamboo basket and place the basket on the pan.

4. Cover the bowls with some baking paper and the lid. Cook for 15 minutes

5. Roast the sesame seeds in a pan.

6. Season the eggs with the seeds and some minced green onion.

Nutrition:

Calories: 13

Fat: 8

Fiber: 12

Carbs: 21

Protein: 5

2. Matcha Mint Iced Tea

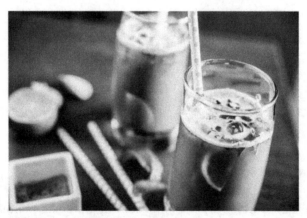

Preparation time: 5 minutes

Cooking Time: 5 minutes

Servings: 3

Ingredients:

- 4 Tbsp. of green Matcha tea ceremonial grade

- 1 lemon fresh juice

- 4 fresh mint twigs

- 4 cups of water

Directions:

1. Put the green tea in a glass, add a little bit of water and mix with milk frothier or a chosen.

2. Pour the tea in an airtight jar and add the lemon juice and the fresh mint. Add the remaining water and stir.

3. Let it rest until cold.

Nutrition:

Calories: 32

Fat: 5

Fiber: 2

Carbs: 11

Protein: 4

3. Coconut Truffles

Preparation time: 1 hour

Cooking Time: 20 minutes

Servings: 14 truffles

Ingredients:

- 1 cup of grated coconut

- 4 Tbsp. of almonds

- 4 Tbsp. of cashews

- 4 Tbsp. of walnuts

- 1 Tbsp. of honey

- 1/4 tsp. of vanilla powder

- 1 Tbsp. of coconut milk

- 3 Tbsp. of coconut oil

- 14 almonds

- Grated coconut for decoration

Directions:

1. In a mixer mix the almonds, the cashews, the walnuts and the grated coconut. (Keep 14 almonds for the filling).

2. Add the coconut oil, the honey, the vanilla powder and the coconut milk and mix again.

3. Shape 15 grams balls, and fill each of them with 1 almond.

4. Roll them into the grated coconut and refrigerate for 1 hour.

Nutrition:

Calories: 13

Fat: 15

Fiber: 6

Carbs: 15

Protein: 3

4. Soft Strawberry Cake

Preparation time: 15 minutes

Cooking time: 45 minutes

Servings: 6

Ingredients:

- 1 cup of almonds flour

- 1/3 cup of arrowroot

- 4 eggs

- 1/2 lb. of strawberries

- 3 Tbsp. of honey

- 1/4 tsp. of vanilla powder

- 1 tsp. of baking soda

- Salt

- 5 Tbsp. of ghee

Directions:

1. Beat the eggs together with the honey, add the heated ghee.

2. In another bowl mix almond flour, vanilla powder, baking soda, arrowroot and salt.

3. Mix the two compounds together.

4. Cut the strawberries into 4 pieces.

5. Pour the compound in a baking tin covered with some baking paper, add the strawberries.

6. Cook in the oven for 45 minutes (330F).

Nutrition:

Calories: 43

Fat: 17

Fiber: 8

Carbs: 21

Protein: 7

5.   Chestnuts And Walnuts Cookies

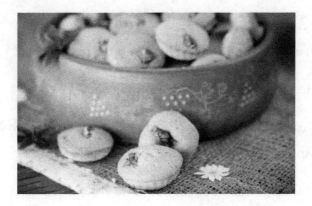

Preparation time: 10 minutes

Cooking time: 20 minutes

Servings: 13 cookies

Ingredients:

- 1 cup of chestnuts flour

- 1/2 cup of walnuts flour

- 1 egg

- 3 Tbsp. of coconut sugar

- 1/2 tsp. of baking soda

- 3 Tbsp. of ghee

- 13 walnuts (for decoration)

Directions:

1. Mix the dry ingredients in a bowl.

2. In another bowl mix the egg with the heated ghee.

3. Mix the two bowls compound together.

4. Shape 13 balls and put them in baking tin covered with baking paper.

5. Place one walnut on top of every ball and cook in the oven for 20 minutes (330F).

Nutrition:

Calories: 13

Fat: 21

Fiber: 14

Carbs: 32

Protein: 9

6. Avocado, Chocolate And Orange Mousse

Preparation time: 75 minutes

Cooking Time: 20 minutes

Servings: 3

Ingredients:

- 1 avocado

- 3 Tbsp. of cocoa powder

- 1 orange

- 1 Tbsp. of honey

Directions:

1. Cut in half the orange. Squeeze one half and cut in pieces the other one.

2. In a mixer mix the avocado pulp, cocoa powder, honey, 3 Tbsp. of orange juice.

3. Place the mixture in some cups and set in the fridge for 1 hour.

4. Decorate with the orange's pieces.

Nutrition:

Calories: 32

Fat: 5

Fiber: 2

Carbs: 11

Protein: 4

7. Spinach Crepes

Preparation time: 10 minutes

Cooking time: 10 minutes

Servings: 6 crepes

Ingredients:

- 1/4 lb. of spinach

- 3 eggs

- 2 Tbsp. of coconut flour

- 1 Tbsp. of arrowroot flour

- 1/3 cup of coconut milk

- 1/4 cup of water

- Salt

- Coconut oil

Directions:

1. Mix all the ingredients out of the coconut oil in a mixer-.

2. Grease a pan with some coconut oil; put 3 tbsp. of the compound. Cook for 1 minute then turn the crepe.

3. Repeat with the remaining mixture.

Nutrition:

Calories: 31

Fat: 12

Fiber: 7

Carbs: 21

Protein: 8

LUNCH

8. Pumpkin And Bean Vegetables

Preparation time: 10 minutes

Cooking time: 15 minutes

Servings: 4

Ingredients:

- 500 g nutmeg squash

- 1 onion

- 2 cloves of garlic

- 1 tbsp. olive oil

- 1 tbsp. butter

- salt and pepper

- 1 teaspoon turmeric

- 1 teaspoon ground cumin

- 1 teaspoon hot paprika powder

- 150 ml vegetable stock

- 400 g green beans

- 1 tbsp. lemon juice

Directions:

1. Remove the seeds from the pumpkin, remove the skin, cut into wedges, then cut into cubes one to two centimeters in size. Skin and finely dice the onion and garlic.

2. Bring the oil and butter to temperature in a pan. Sauté the onions until translucent over medium heat. Add the garlic and pumpkin, sauté for three minutes, salt and pepper. Dust with the turmeric, cumin and paprika powder. Deglaze with the broth and simmer covered for a quarter of an hour over medium heat.

3. Meanwhile, clean the beans, cut them in half and blanch them in boiling salted water for about five to seven minutes, drain, rinse and drain.

4. Mix the beans with the pumpkin vegetables and cook for two to three minutes. Season the vegetables with lemon juice, salt and pepper.

Nutrition:

Calories: 21

Fat: 4

Fiber: 2

Carbs: 11

Protein: 4

9. Wok Vegetables With Tofu

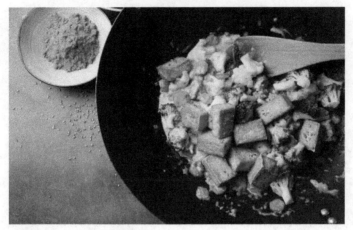

Preparation time: 10 minutes

Cooking time: 15 minutes

Servings: 4

Ingredients:

- 1 organic lemon

- 8 stalks of mint

- 3 centimeters of fresh ginger

- 1 red chili pepper

- 4 tbsp. neutral oil

- salt

- 400 g broad green beans

- 2 red peppers

- 2 spring onions

- 400 g tofu

- 150 ml vegetable stock, instant

Directions:

1. Wash and dry the lemon, rub the peel. Clean and dry the mint and remove the leaves. Remove the peel from the ginger and cut. Clean the chili pepper, remove the seeds. Finely chop the mint, ginger and chili. Mix with the zest of the lemon, a tablespoon of oil and the salt.

2. Clean the beans and remove the end pieces, cut the beans diagonally into pieces just under one centimeter wide. Boil enough water in a saucepan, season with salt and boil the beans for about two minutes. Pour into a sieve, pour cold water over it and allow draining. Clean the peppers, cut into quarters and remove the seeds and the walls. Cut the quarters of the peppers into strips. Set and wash the spring onions and cut into rings. Drain the tofu and dice it an inch.

3. Bring the wok to temperature and add oil. Add the tofu, season with salt and fry for about four minutes until crispy. Add the vegetables and onions and stir-fry for about three minutes. Fry the herb paste, add the stock and season with

salt. Serve the vegetables immediately. Rice or Asian noodles go well with it.

Nutrition:

Calories: 43

Fat: 11

Fiber: 8

Carbs: 21

Protein: 5

10. Pumpkin And Mushroom Curry

Preparation time: 10 minutes

Cooking time: 15 minutes

Servings: 2

Ingredients:

- 0.5 Hokkaido pumpkin (400 g)

- 250 g small mushrooms

- 1 onion

- 2 inches of ginger

- 2 tbsp. neutral oil

- 1 teaspoon curry paste, red or green

- 200 ml coconut milk

- 50 ml of water

- salt

- 2 teaspoons of lime juice, alternatively lemon juice

- 0.25 frets

- coriander

Directions:

1. Clean the pumpkin and scrape out the seeds and fibrous pulp. Cut the pumpkin with the skin into pieces about two centimeters in size. Clean the mushrooms, rub them with a clean cloth and, depending on the size, leave them whole or cut in half. Remove the skin from the onion and ginger and cut into cubes.

2. Bring the oil to temperature in a saucepan and fry the mushrooms over medium heat. Add the pieces of pumpkin and fry briefly. Add the onion and ginger.

3. Mix the curry paste into the vegetables and fry briefly. Pour in the coconut milk and about 60 ml of water. Season the dish with salt and the juice of the lime and cook covered.

4. Meanwhile, clean and dry the coriander, remove the leaves and chop up. Flavor the curry with salt and sprinkle with the coriander.

Nutrition:

Calories: 15

Fat: 5

Fiber: 13

Carbs: 23

Protein: 3

11. Herbal Frittata With Peppers And Feta

Preparation time: 10 minutes

Cooking time: 15 minutes

Servings: 4

Ingredients:

- 5 eggs

- sea-salt

- 1 bunch of parsley

- 4 tbsp. freshly grated parmesan

- 2 red peppers

- 1 yellow pepper

- 150 g feta

- 3 tbsp. olive oil

- salt and pepper

Directions:

1. Mix the eggs in a bowl with a pinch of sea salt. Clean and dry the parsley, peel off the leaves and chop. Stir the parsley and parmesan into the eggs. Divide the peppers lengthways, clean, wash and cut into strips. Crumble the feta.

2. Bring the olive oil to temperature in a pan. Add the paprika strips and steam for about two minutes, season with a little salt and pepper. Stream the egg mixture over it and spread the feta on top. Cover and let the frittata stand for six to eight minutes over a moderate heat. Slide on a platter, cut into pieces and serve warm or cold.

Nutrition:

Calories: 32

Fat: 5

Fiber: 2

Carbs: 11

Protein: 4

12. Vegetable Coconut Curry

Preparation time: 10 minutes

Cooking time: 20 minutes

Servings: 4

Ingredients:

- 300 g pointed cabbage

- 300 g Swiss chard

- 300 g broccoli

- 2 spring onions

- 4 centimeters of fresh ginger

- 4 stalks of basil

- 1 organic lime

- 2 tbsp. neutral oil

- salt

- 1 teaspoon of red or green curry paste

- 400 g coconut milk, pack or can

Directions:

1. Clean the vegetable parts. Cut the strong ribs flatter in the middle of the pointed cabbage. Cut the cabbage and the chard

into strips one centimeter wide. Divide the broccoli, peel the stem and cut into slices about five millimeters thick.

2. Set and wash the spring onions and cut into rings. Remove the peel from the ginger and cut it first into slices, then into fine strips. Clean and dry the basil, peel off the leaves and chop. Wash the lime with hot water and dry, rub the peel and squeeze out the juice.

3. Set the oil to temperature in a large pan. Pour in the vegetables, add a little salt and fry over high to medium heat for three to four minutes until al dente. Attach the spring onions and ginger and fry. Stir in the curry paste. Pour in the coconut milk and bring to the boil once.

4. Season the curry with the peel of the lime, two to three tablespoons of lime juice and a little salt. Sprinkle with the basil and serve. It is best to serve fragrant rice and a cucumber salad.

Nutrition:

Calories: 12

Fat: 11

Fiber: 9

Carbs: 25

Protein: 4

13. Wok Ratatouille

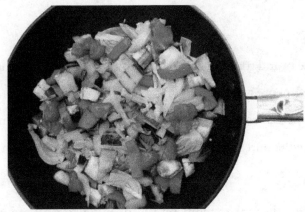

Preparation time: 10 minutes

Cooking time: 15 minutes

Servings: 2

Ingredients:

- 1 zucchini (200 g)

- 0.5 small eggplants (150 g)

- 1 red pepper

- 100 g cherry tomatoes

- 4 sprigs of thyme

- 1 sprig of rosemary

- 2 cloves of garlic

- 3 tbsp. olive oil

- salt and pepper

Directions:

1. Clean and trim the vegetables. Cut the zucchini, aborigine and bell pepper separately into half a centimeter cubes. Cut the tomatoes in half. Clean and dry the herbs and remove the needles and leaves and chop. Remove the garlic from the skin and cut into cubes.

2. Bring the wok to temperature and add two tablespoons of oil. Fry the eggplant cubes over high heat for two to three minutes while stirring. Add the zucchini and bell pepper with the remaining oil and herbs and stir-fry all ingredients for another two to three minutes.

3. Mix in the tomatoes and garlic and fry briefly. Season the dish with salt and pepper and serve immediately. Fresh baguette is served with it.

Nutrition:

Calories: 13

Fat: 21

Fiber: 14

Carbs: 32

Protein: 9

14. Tofu With Curry Mushrooms

Preparation time: 10 minutes

Cooking time: 20 minutes

Servings: 4

Ingredients:

- 500 g mushrooms, or Egerlinge

- 2 spring onions

- 2 cloves of garlic

- 0.5 frets of parsley

- 0.5 organic lemon

- 2 teaspoons of coriander seeds

- 4 tbsp. neutral oil

- 2 teaspoons of hot curry powder

- 200 ml plant cream, preferably almond or oat cream

- salt and pepper

- 500 g tofu

Directions:

1. Rub the mushrooms with kitchen paper and remove the ends of the stems. Cut the mushrooms into slices. Clean and clean the spring onions and cut into rings.

2. Remove the garlic from the skin and cut into thin slices. Clean, dry and finely chop the parsley. Wash and dry half of the lemon with hot water, finely grate the peel, squeeze out a tablespoon of juice.

3. Heat a large saucepan. Roast the coriander in it for about a minute while stirring, then remove and finely pound in a mortar.

4. Bring two tablespoons of oil to temperature in the saucepan. In it, stir-fry the mushrooms over high heat for about four minutes until the liquid has evaporated again. Attach the onions and garlic and fry briefly. Dust the curry powder over it, also fry a little. Set in the cream and bring to the boil. Season the mushrooms with the coriander, lemon zest and lemon juice, salt and pepper to taste, then keep warm.

5. Slice the tofu into thin slices and season with salt and pepper to taste. Heat the remaining oil in a large pan. Attach the tofu slices and fry for about four minutes on each side over high heat. Mix the parsley with the mushrooms. Serve with the tofu.

Nutrition:

Calories: 21

Fat: 13

Fiber: 5

Carbs: 10

Protein: 9

15. Baked Zucchini Fries

Preparation time: 15 minutes

Cooking time: 25 minutes

Servings: 4-6

Ingredients:

- 2 large zucchini

- 1/2 cup almond flour

- 11/2 teaspoons garlic powder

- 11/2 teaspoons onion powder

- 2 eggs, whisked

- Salt

- Freshly ground black pepper

Directions:

1. Preheat the oven to 400F.

2. Chop the ends off the zucchini, and cut them in half widthwise, then lengthwise. Cut into French fry–like strips, and pat dry with a paper towel.

3. In a bowl, merge together the almond flour, garlic powder, and onion powder. Dip the zucchini fries in the egg, let any excess egg drip off, and toss them in the almond flour mixture. Season with salt and pepper.

4. Set the fries out on a baking sheet, put them in the oven, and immediately lower the heat to 350F. Cook until the fries are crisp, checking on them halfway through the cooking time and lowering the heat if they're getting brown too quickly.

5. Serve immediately.

Nutrition:

Calories: 40

Fat: 6g

Carbs: 20g

Protein: 2g

Fiber: 1g

Sugar: 1g

16. Pad Thai

Preparation time: 10 minutes

Cooking time: 20 minutes

Servings: 4

Ingredients:

- 1 pound boneless skinless chicken breast

- 2 tablespoons coconut aminos

- 2 garlic cloves, minced

- 1 teaspoon grated fresh ginger

- 1 to 2 tablespoons almond butter

- 1 tablespoon freshly squeezed lime juice, plus 4 lime wedges for garnish

- 2 teaspoons fish sauce

- 1/2 teaspoon red pepper

- 2 large zucchini, spiralized or julienned into noodles

- 1 cup bean sprouts

- 1/3 cup slivered almonds

- 2 to 3 tablespoons chopped fresh cilantro, for garnish

Directions:

1. Set a pot of water, boil or steam the chicken breasts for about 15 minutes, or until they're cooked through. Pat dry and slice into bite-size pieces.

2. In a large bowl, mix the coconut aminos, garlic, ginger, almond butter, lime juice, fish sauce, and red pepper flakes. Set aside.

3. Set a large skillet over medium-low heat, gently sauté the zucchini until they just start to become tender. Detach from the heat, and mix in with the pad thai sauce. Stir in the chicken, and serve topped with bean sprouts, almonds, cilantro, and a wedge of lime.

Nutrition

Calories: 150

Fat: 12g

Carbs: 9g

Protein: 24g

Fiber: 6g

Sugar: 0g

17. Zucchini-Spinach Fritters

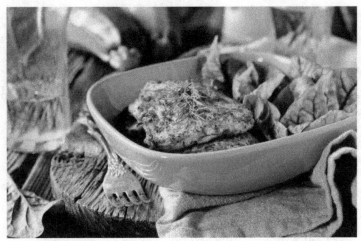

Preparation time: 5 minutes

Cooking time: 15 minutes

Servings: 4-6

Ingredients:

- 1 (14-ounce) can artichoke hearts, clear and chopped

- 12 ounces fresh spinach, washed, cooked, and drained

- 1 large zucchini, shredded

- 6 scallions, chopped

- 2 or 3 garlic cloves, minced

- 2 eggs, lightly beaten

- 1/2 cup almond flour

- 1 teaspoon salt

- 1 tablespoon extra-virgin olive oil

Directions:

1. With your hands, press as much liquid out of the artichoke hearts, spinach, and zucchini as possible.

2. In a food processor, merge the artichoke hearts, spinach, zucchini, scallions, and garlic until roughly chopped. Set the mixture to a large bowl, add the eggs and almond flour, and season with salt. Mix well.

3. Set a large nonstick sauté pan over medium-high heat, heat the olive oil. Drop heaping tablespoons of the mixture into the pan, and cook for 2 to 3 minutes on each side, flattening them a little with your spatula to make them into mini-pancake shapes.

4. Serve immediately.

Nutrition:

Calories: 21

Fat: 4

Fiber: 2

Carbs: 11

Protein: 4

18. Emergency Pasta With Zoodles

Preparation time: 5 minutes

Cooking time: 5 minutes

Servings: 4

Ingredients:

- 1/4 cup extra-virgin olive oil

- 2 or 3 garlic cloves, thinly sliced

- 1/4 hot red pepper, minced (or 1/4 teaspoon red pepper flakes)

- 3 or 4 large zucchini, spiralized or julienned into noodles

- Salt

- Freshly ground black pepper

Directions:

1. In a large sauté pan over medium-low heat, heat the olive oil. Add the garlic, and stir it around. Detach from the heat as soon as the garlic becomes fragrant—about 30 seconds—because you don't want to burn it at all. Add the hot red pepper, and pour the sauce into a serving dish.

2. In the same pan over medium heat, sauté the zucchini noodles for 3 to 4 minutes, just until slightly softened. Transfer the

noodles to the serving dish, season with salt and pepper, and toss with the sauce.

3. Serve immediately.

Nutrition:

Calories: 32

Fat: 3 g

Carbs: 12 g

Protein: 1 g

Fiber: 3 g

Sugar: 1.9 g

19. Zucchini Lasagna

Preparation time: 15 minutes

Cooking time: 1 hour and 15 minutes

Servings: 6-8

Ingredients:

- 2 large zucchini

- 1 pound spicy Italian sausage

- 1 pound ground beef

- 1 onion, diced

- 1 small green bell pepper, diced

- 1 (16-ounce) can tomato sauce

- 1 cup tomato paste

- 1/4 cup red wine (optional; omit if strict Paleo)

- 2 tablespoons chopped fresh basil

- 2 tablespoons chopped fresh parsley

- 1 tablespoon chopped fresh oregano

- Salt

- Freshly ground black pepper

- 1 pound fresh mushrooms, sliced

Directions:

1. Preheat the oven to 325F.

2. With a vegetable peeler to cut the zucchini lengthwise into small, thin sheets that resemble lasagna.

3. Set a large skillet; cook the Italian sausage for 5 to 7 minutes per side, until browned. Remove from the skillet, and set aside. Attach the ground beef to the skillet, and cook for 5 minutes, using a wooden spoon to break up the beef. Attach

the onion and bell pepper, and continue cooking until the beef is no longer pink, about another 5 minutes.

4. Whip in the tomato sauce, tomato paste, wine (if using), basil, parsley, and oregano, and season with salt and pepper. Once the sauce begins to boil, lessen the heat and simmer for 20 minutes, stirring frequently. Remove from the heat.

5. To assemble the lasagna, start by spreading half the meat sauce into the bottom of an 8-by-12-inch baking dish. Layer half the zucchini slices over the meat sauce. Add the Italian sausage and all the mushrooms. Continue layering the lasagna by adding the remaining meat sauce and zucchini sheets.

6. Seal with foil, and bake the lasagna for 45 minutes. Carefully remove the foil, raise the oven temperature to 375F, and bake for an additional 10 to 15 minutes.

7. Detach from the oven and allow to rest for 5 minutes before slicing. Serve warm.

Nutrition:

Calories: 21

Fat: 4 g

Carbs: 14 g

Protein: 3.1 g

Fiber: 2.7 g

Sugar: 2.9 g

20. Zucchini-Noodle Ramen

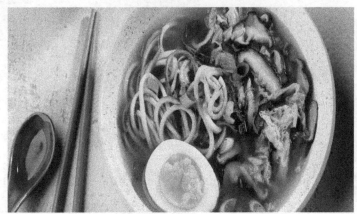

Preparation time: 15 minutes

Cooking time: 2 hours and 15 minutes

Servings: 4-6

Ingredients:

- 1 pound pork tenderloin

- 1 tablespoon salt

- 2 bunches scallions, divided

- 1 (1-inch) piece fresh ginger root, sliced

- 4 garlic cloves, crushed

- Toppings (optional): hardboiled eggs, kimchi, jalapeño peppers, fresh cilantro

- 5 tablespoons coconut aminos

- 2 tablespoons sake (optional; omit if strict Paleo)

- 11/2 tablespoons sesame oil

- 4 large zucchini, spiralized or julienned

Directions:

1. Season the pork with the salt, and refrigerate overnight.

2. Remove the pork from the refrigerator, and place in a large saucepan over medium-high heat. Add 11/2 bunches of scallions and the ginger and garlic to the pan with enough water to just cover the pork. Set to a boil, lower the heat, and simmer for at least 2 hours (although longer is better, if possible).

3. While the broth is cooking, prepare all your toppings (if using): Soft-boil the eggs (see here), slice the jalapeños and the remaining 1/2 bunch of scallions, and chop the cilantro.

4. Add the coconut aminos, sake (if using), and sesame oil to the broth. Continue to simmer, and add the zucchini noodles about 5 minutes before you're ready to serve.

5. Transfer the pork to a platter, slice it, and transfer it back to the saucepan. Serve the ramen with whichever toppings sound good to you.

Nutrition:

Calories: 21

Fat: 5 g

Carbs: 11 g

Protein: 1 g

Fiber: 5 g

Sugar: 0.3 g

21. Stuffed Zucchini Boats

Preparation time: 10 minutes

Cooking time: 1 hour

Servings: 4

Ingredients:

- 4 large zucchini

- 1 pound ground beef

- 2 tablespoons extra-virgin olive oil

- 1 onion, diced

- 2 garlic cloves, chopped

- Salt

- Freshly ground black pepper

- 3/4 cup green olives, roughly chopped

- 2 hardboiled eggs, chopped

Directions:

1. Preheat the oven to 350F.

2. Cut the zucchini lengthwise, and scoop the insides out with a spoon. Chop the inside parts, and add them to a medium bowl with the ground beef.

3. In a skillet over medium-high warmth, heat the olive oil. Sauté the onion and garlic until the onion is slightly translucent, about 5 minutes. Add the ground beef–zucchini mixture, and cook for about 5 minutes more, until completely browned, breaking the meat up as you cook it. Season with salt and pepper.

4. Detach the skillet from the heat, and add the olives and hardboiled eggs. Stir well.

5. Stuff the zucchini boats with the meat mixture, and place them on a baking sheet. Bake for 45 minutes, until tender, and serve.

Nutrition:

Calories: 17

Fat: 5 g

Carbs: 12 g

Protein: 1 g

Fiber: 3 g

Sugar: 1.3 g

22. Stuffed Squash

Preparation time: 10 minutes

Cooking time: 1 hour

Servings: 2

Ingredients:

- 2 round squash, such as acorn or 8-ball zucchini

- 2 tablespoons extra-virgin olive oil

- Salt

- Freshly ground black pepper

- 1/2 teaspoon onion powder

- 1/2 onion, diced

- 1 pound ground beef

- 11/2 teaspoons garlic powder

- 11/2 teaspoons dried oregano

- 1/8 teaspoon red pepper flakes

- 1 (14.5-ounce) can diced tomatoes, drained

- 1 or 2 tablespoons chopped fresh basil or oregano

Directions:

1. Preheat the oven to 350F.

2. Carefully cut the tops off the squash, scoop out the seeds, trim the bottoms if necessary so they will stand up straight, and season the insides with the olive oil, salt, pepper, and onion powder. Roast for 45 minutes.

3. While the squash are in the oven, in a large sauté pan over medium heat, sauté the onion until slightly translucent, about 5 minutes. Add the beef, and break it up with a wooden spoon. Season with the garlic powder, oregano, red pepper flakes, and some more salt and pepper.

4. Once the beef is no longer pink, 7 to 8 minutes, reduce the heat to low and add the tomatoes. Continue to simmer until the squash have finished cooking.

5. To serve, place each squash in a bowl or on a plate and spoon the beef mixture into the centers. Garnish with the basil.

Nutrition:

Calories: 213

Fat: 3 g

Carbs: 9 g

Protein: 3 g

Fiber: 2.1 g

Sugar: 3 g

23. Red Salsa

Preparation Time: 35 Minutes

Cooking Time: 15 Minutes

Servings: 8

Ingredients:

- 4 Roma tomatoes, halved

- 1/4 cup chopped cilantro

- 1 jalapeno pepper, deseeded, halved

- 1/2 of a medium white onion, peeled, cut into quarters

- 3 cloves of garlic, peeled

- 1/2 teaspoon salt

- 1 tablespoon brown sugar

- 1 teaspoon apple cider vinegar

Directions:

1. Switch on the oven, then set it to 425 degrees F and let it preheat.

2. Meanwhile, take a baking sheet, line it with foil, and then spread tomato, jalapeno pepper, onion, and garlic.

3. Bake the vegetables for 15 minutes until vegetables have cooked and begin to brown and then let the vegetables cool for 3 minutes.

4. Transfer the roasted vegetables into a blender, add remaining ingredients and then pulse until smooth.

5. Tip the salsa into a medium bowl and then chill it for 30 minutes before serving with vegetable sticks.

Nutrition:

Calories: 240

Fat: 0 g

Protein: 0 g

Carbs: 48 g

Fiber: 16 g

24. Pinto Bean Dip

Preparation Time: 5 Minutes

Cooking Time: 0 Minutes

Servings: 4

Ingredients:

- 15 ounces canned pinto beans

- 1 jalapeno pepper

- 2 teaspoons ground cumin

- 3 tablespoons nutritional yeast

- 1/3 cup basil salsa

Directions:

1. Merge all the ingredients in a food processor, cover with the lid, and then pulse until smooth.

2. Tip the dip in a bowl and then serve with vegetable slices.

Nutrition:

Calories: 360

Fat: 0 g

Protein: 24 g

Carbs: 72 g

Fiber: 24 g

25. Smoky Red Pepper Hummus

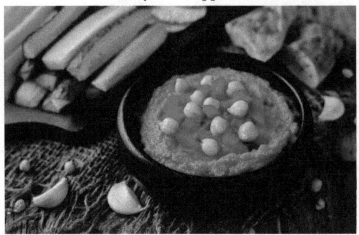

Preparation Time: 5 Minutes

Cooking Time: 0 Minutes

Servings: 4

Ingredients:

- 1/4 cup roasted red peppers

- 1 cup cooked chickpeas

- 1/8 teaspoon garlic powder

- 1/2 teaspoon salt

- 1/8 teaspoon ground black pepper

- 1/4 teaspoon ground cumin

- 1/4 teaspoon red chili powder

- 1 tablespoon Tahini

- 2 tablespoons water

Directions:

1. Set all the ingredients in the jar of the food processor and then pulse until smooth.

2. Tip the hummus in a bowl and then serve with vegetable slices.

Nutrition:

Calories: 489

Fat: 30 g

Protein: 9 g

Carbs: 15 g

Fiber: 6 g

26. Spinach Dip

Preparation Time: 20 Minutes

Cooking Time: 5 Minutes

Servings: 8

Ingredients:

- 3/4 cup cashews

- 3.5ounces soft tofu

- 6 ounces of spinach leaves

- 1 medium white onion, peeled, diced

- 2 teaspoons minced garlic

- 1/2 teaspoon salt

- 3 tablespoons olive oil

Directions:

1. Set cashews in a bowl, cover with hot water, and then let them soak for 15 minutes.

2. After 15 minutes, drain the cashews and then set aside until required.

3. Take a medium skillet pan, add oil to it and then place the pan

4. Set the onion, and cook until tender, stir in garlic and then continue cooking for 30 seconds until fragrant.

5. Scoop the onion mixture into a blender, add remaining ingredients and then pulse until smooth.

6. Tip the dip into a bowl and then serve with chips.

Nutrition:

Calories: 134.6

Fat: 8.6 g

Protein: 10 g

Carbs: 6.3 g

Fiber: 1.4 g

27. Tomatillo Salsa

Preparation Time: 5 Minutes

Cooking Time: 20 Minutes

Servings: 8

Ingredients:

- 5 medium tomatillos, chopped

- 3 cloves of garlic, peeled, chopped

- 3 Roma tomatoes, chopped

- 1 jalapeno, chopped

- 1/2 of a medium red onion, skinned, chopped

- 1 Anaheim chili

- 2 teaspoons salt

- 1 teaspoon ground cumin

- 1 lime, juiced

- 1/4 cup cilantro leaves

- 3/4 cup of water

Directions:

1. Take a medium pot, place it over medium heat, pour in water, and then add onion, tomatoes, tomatillo, jalapeno, and Anaheim chili.

2. Sauté the vegetables for 15 minutes, remove the pot from heat, add cilantro and lime juice and then stir in salt.

3. Remove pot from heat and then pulse by using an immersion blender until smooth.

4. Serve the salsa with chips.

Nutrition:

Calories: 317.4

Fat: 0 g

Protein: 16 g

Carbs: 64 g

Fiber: 16 g

28. Arugula Pesto Couscous

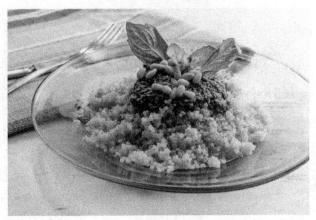

Preparation Time: 10 Minutes

Cooking Time: 20 Minutes

Servings: 4

Ingredients:

- 8 ounces Israeli couscous

- 3 large tomatoes, chopped

- 3 cups arugula leaves

- 1/2 cup parsley leaves

- 6 cloves of garlic, peeled

- 1/2 cup walnuts

- 3/4 teaspoon salt

- 1 cup and 1 tablespoon olive oil

- 2 cups vegetable broth

Directions:

1. Take a medium saucepan, place it over medium-high heat, add 1 tablespoon oil and then let it heat.

2. Add couscous, stir until mixed, and then cook for 4 minutes until fragrant and toasted.

3. Pour in the broth, stir until mixed, bring it to a boil, switch heat to medium level and then simmer for 12 minutes until the couscous has absorbed all the liquid and turn tender.

4. When done, remove the pan from heat, fluff it with a fork, and then set aside until required.

5. While couscous cooks, prepare the pesto, and for this, place walnuts in a blender, add garlic, and then pulse until nuts have broken.

6. Add arugula, parsley, and salt, pulse until well combined, and then blend in oil until smooth.

7. Transfer couscous to a salad bowl, add tomatoes and prepared pesto, and then toss until mixed.

8. Serve straight away.

Nutrition:

Calories: 73

Fat: 4 g

Protein: 2 g

Carbs: 8 g

Fiber: 2 g

29. Oatmeal And Raisin Balls

Preparation Time: 40 Minutes

Cooking Time: 0 Minutes

Servings: 4

Ingredients:

- 1 cup rolled oats

- 1/4 cup raisins

- 1/2 cup peanut butter

Directions:

1. Place oats in a large bowl, add raisins and peanut butter, and then stir until well combined.

2. Shape the mixture into twelve balls, 1 tablespoon of mixture per ball, and then arrange the balls on a sheet.

3. Set the baking sheet into the freezer for 30 minutes until firm and then serve.

Nutrition:

Calories: 135

Fat: 6 g

Protein: 8 g

Carbs: 13 g

Fiber: 4 g

30. Paleo Sweet Potato Tater Tots

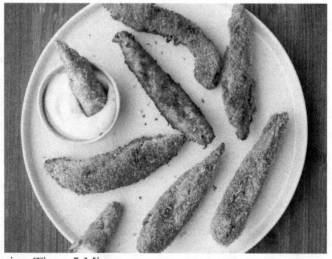

Preparation Time: 5 Minutes

Cooking Time: 20 Minutes

Servings: 4

Ingredients:

- 2 Large Sweet Potatoes (Skinned and Roughly Cubed)

- 1/4 Medium Finely Diced Onion

- 2 tablespoons of Coconut Flour

- 1 teaspoon of Garlic Powder

- 1 teaspoon of Chili Powder

- 1/2 teaspoon of Salt

- 1/4 teaspoon of Freshly Ground Pepper

- 1/2 cup of Coconut Oil (For Frying)

Directions:

1. Bring your large-sized pot of water to a boil. Add your sweet potatoes and cook for approximately 5 minutes. Drain and rinse with cold water. Shake off any excess water.

2. Place your sweet potato and onion into your food processor and pulse to break down into smaller pieces. Transfer to a large-sized bowl. Stir in your coconut flour, chili powder, garlic powder, salt, and pepper. Stir well to combine.

3. With your hands to shape the potato mixture into small cylinders. Place to the side until ready to fry.

4. Warmth your coconut oil in a heavy skillet until hot. Working in batches, add your tater tots to the skillet and fry until golden brown.

5. Serve and Enjoy!

Nutrition:

Calories: 301

Fat: 9.3 g;

Protein: 6.8 g

Carbs: 49 g

Fiber: 1.9

31. Ropa Vieja

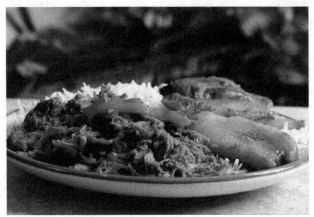

Preparation time: 10 minutes

Cooking time: 1 hour and 20 minutes

Servings: 4

Ingredients:

- 1 to 2 tablespoons extra-virgin olive oil

- 2 to 3 pounds flank steak

- 1 red onion, sliced

- 4 garlic cloves, minced

- 2 red bell peppers, cut into strips

- 2 green bell peppers, cut into strips

- 1 teaspoon dried oregano

- 1 teaspoon ground cumin

- 1/4 cup sherry vinegar

- 3 cups beef broth

- 1 tablespoon tomato paste

- 2 dried bay leaves

- Salt

- Freshly ground black pepper

- 1/2 cup chopped fresh cilantro

Directions:

1. In an oven or pot over medium-high heat, warmth the olive oil. Brown the beef (you may need to cut it in half and work in batches), about 3 minutes per side. Set aside.

2. Set the heat to medium, and attach the onion, garlic, and red and green bell peppers to the pot. Stirring frequently, cook for 5 to 7 minutes, until tender. Add the oregano and cumin, and cook for 1 minute more.

3. Attach the sherry vinegar, and deglaze the pan, stirring up any browned bits from the bottom. Cook. Add the broth and tomato paste, and stir well to combine. Set in the bay leaves, and return the beef to the pot. Season with salt and pepper.

Bring the whole thing to a simmer, reduce the heat to low, and cook for another hour.

4. Set the meat to a platter, and shred it. Serve garnished with the cilantro.

Nutrition:

Calories: 32

Fat: 5

Fiber: 2

Carbs: 11

Protein: 4

32. Vaca Frita

Preparation time: 10 minutes

Cooking time: 1 hour

Servings: 4

Ingredients:

- 2 pounds flank steak

- 1 dried bay leaf

- 2 onions, 1 quartered and the other sliced

- 2 tablespoons grass-fed butter

- 2 garlic cloves, smashed

- 1/4 cup freshly squeezed lime juice,

- 3 to 4 tablespoons extra-virgin olive oil,

- Salt

- Freshly ground black pepper

Directions:

1. In a large pot, cover the flank steak (you may need to cut it in half or even quarters), bay leaf, and quartered onion with enough water to cover the meat by an inch. Set to a boil, and then simmer over low heat for 20 minutes.

2. While the beef is cooking, in a medium skillet over medium-low heat, heat the butter. Gently cook the sliced onion until it is very soft and dark brown, about 20 minutes.

3. When the beef finishes cooking, transfer it to a platter and allow it to cool before using your hands to shred it into very thin pieces.

4. Transfer the shredded beef to a large bowl, and add the garlic and lime juice. Mix well, and then allow it to marinate for 30 minutes on the counter.

5. In a large skillet over high heat, heat 1 tablespoon of olive oil. Working in batches, fry the shredded beef in a single layer

until very browned and crispy, 4 to 7 minutes per batch. Flavor with salt and pepper, and remove from the heat. Repeat with the rest of the beef, adding more oil as necessary.

6. Serve each plate of vaca frita topped with some of the sautéed onions and a wedge of fresh lime.

Nutrition:

Calories 119

Fat 8.1

Fiber 1.4

Carbs 11.1

Protein 3

33. Steak Marsala

Preparation time: 10 minutes

Cooking time: 35 minutes

Servings: 4

Ingredients:

For The Sauce

- 3 tablespoons extra-virgin olive oil

- 1/2 onion, sliced

- 10 ounces mushrooms

- 2 garlic cloves, minced

- 1/2 cup Marsala wine

- 11/2 cups beef broth

- Salt

- Freshly ground black pepper

For The Steaks

- 4 large steaks (rib eyes or sirloin)

- 4 tablespoons grass-fed butter

Directions:

To Make the Sauce

1. In a medium saucepan over medium heat, warmth the olive oil. Sauté the onion until slightly translucent, about 5 minutes. Attach the mushrooms and garlic, and cook for another 5 minutes.

2. Add the Marsala wine, and deglaze the pan, scraping up any browned bits from the bottom, and add the beef broth. Flavor with salt and pepper, and cook down until the sauce begins to thicken, 8 to 10 minutes. Set the heat to low, and simmer until ready to serve.

To Cook the Steaks

1. Preheat the oven to 400F.

2. In a ovenproof skillet over high heat, sear the steaks for 2 to 3 minutes per side, until browned. Set to the oven, and cook for 6 to 10 minutes, depending on how rare you want them. Remove from the oven, and place 1 tablespoon of butter on each steak.

3. Let rest for 10 minutes before slicing. Top with the Marsala sauce, and serve.

Nutrition:

Calories: 134.6

Fat: 8.6 g

Protein: 10 g

Carbs: 6.3 g

Fiber: 1.4 g

34. Sausage-Stuffed Dates Wrapped In Bacon

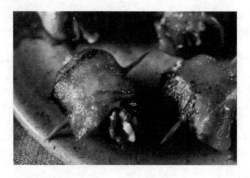

Preparation time: 15 minutes

Cooking time: 30 minutes

Servings: 8-10

Ingredients:

- 16 to 20 dates, pitted

- 1 pound spicy ground pork sausage

- 8 to 10 slices bacon, halved

Directions:

1. Preheat the oven to 400F.

2. Carefully slice each date down the middle

3. Make a roll of sausage in your hands. Stuff each date with a sausage oval. Cover each stuffed date with half a strip of bacon, and set it on a baking sheet.

4. Bake the dates until the bacon is crispy and the sausage is cooked through, and serve.

Nutrition:

Calories: 13

Fat: 9

Fiber: 12

Carbs: 21

Protein: 8

35. Candied Bacon Salad

Preparation time: 5 minutes

Cooking time: 20 minutes

Servings: 4

Ingredients:

- 10 to 12 ounces thick-cut bacon, halved or quartered

- 1/2 cup maple syrup

- 3 to 4 cups field greens (or your favorite salad mix)

- 1/2 cup pecans

- 1/4 cup Apple Cider Vinaigrette (here)

Directions:

1. Preheat the oven to 400F.

2. On a baking sheet, set out the bacon in a single layer, and brush with the maple syrup. Bake until the bacon is as crispy. Chop or crumble the bacon into bite-size pieces.

3. In a large serving bowl, merge the greens with the pecans and Apple Cider Vinaigrette. Top with the candied bacon, and serve.

Nutrition:

Calories 32

Fat 3.5

Fiber 0

Carbs 0.1

Protein 0

36. Sesame Pork Salad

Preparation time: 30 minutes

Cooking time: 10 minutes

Servings: 4

Ingredients:

- 2 tablespoons honey

- 2 tablespoons sesame oil

- 1 tablespoon coconut aminos

- 1/2 tablespoon chili oil

- 1/2 tablespoon fish sauce

- 1/2 onion, diced

- 2 garlic cloves, minced

- 1/4 tsp. freshly ground black pepper

- 1 pound pork cutlets, cut into strips

- 2 to 3 cups chopped romaine (or your favorite salad lettuce)

- 1 or 2 tablespoons sesame seeds, for garnish

Directions:

1. In a large bowl, stir to merge the honey, sesame oil, coconut aminos, chili oil, fish sauce, onion, garlic, and pepper. Attach the pork, and marinate for at least 20 minutes.

2. Warmth a cast iron pan or skillet over high heat. Add the pork, and cook until seared on all sides, about 10 minutes.

3. Put the chopped lettuce in a large serving bowl, and top it with the cooked pork. Garnish with the sesame seeds, and serve.

Nutrition:

Calories 119

Fat 8.1

Fiber 1.4

Carbs 11.1

Protein 3

37. Ground Pork Stir-Fry

Preparation time: 5 minutes

Cooking time: 20 minutes

Servings: 4

Ingredients:

- 1 1/2 tablespoons extra-virgin olive oil or coconut oil

- 1/2 onion, diced

- 1 green bell pepper, cut into strips

- 10 ounces mushrooms, sliced

- 1 or 2 small zucchini, diced

- 3 garlic cloves, minced

- 1 pound ground pork

- Salt

- Freshly ground black pepper

- 1/4 teaspoon red pepper flakes

Directions:

1. Set a frying pan over medium heat, warmth the olive oil. Add the onion, and sauté until slightly translucent, about 5 minutes.

2. Add the bell pepper, mushrooms, and zucchini. Allow to cool down for another 5 minutes before adding the garlic.

3. Move all the sautéed vegetables to the outside edges of the pan, and put the ground pork in the middle. Flavor with salt and pepper, and cook, stirring with a wooden spoon to break up the pieces, until the pork and the garlic begin to brown, about 5 minutes. Stir the vegetables into the center until everything is well mixed. Set the heat up to medium-high, and cook until some of the pork begins to crisp up, about 5 minutes.

4. Add the red pepper flakes, give it another stir, and serve hot.

Nutrition:

Calories: 204

Fat: 1.1 g;

Protein: 6.5 g;

Carbs: 48 g;

Fiber: 8.3 g

38. Green Chile Chicken Breasts With Sauce

Preparation time: 5 minutes

Cooking time: 30 minutes

Servings: 6

Ingredients:

- 1 tablespoon sesame seeds, toasted

- 2 tablespoons whipping cream

- 1 tablespoon canola oil

- 6 chicken breast cutlets or fillets

- 3/4 teaspoon of salt, divided

- 1 clove garlic, thinly sliced

- 3 tablespoons slivered almonds, toasted

- 3 scallions, sliced, separated white and green parts

- 3/4 cup of fresh green chilies, chopped and seeded

- 1/2 cup chicken broth, reduced-sodium

- 2 cups almond milk, unsweetened

Directions

1. In a medium-sized saucepan, mix together green chilies, almond milk, garlic, scallion whites, broth and 1/4 teaspoon salt and bring the mixture to a boil.

2. Then minimize the heat and simmer for about 20-30 minutes, until the mixture is reduced by half.

3. Now set the mixture in a blender or immersion blender until smooth.

4. Using the remaining 1/2 teaspoon of salt, season the chicken and then heat some oil over medium-heat in a large non-skillet.

5. In the skillet, cook half of the chicken for about 1-2 minutes each side, until browned.

6. Then put the first batch of the chicken in the pan and then pour the sauce. Cook at low heat to simmer, for about 4-7 minutes until the chicken is tender and cooked through.

7. When done, remove from heat and then pour the sauce over your chicken.

8. Use the reserved sesame seeds and scallion greens to sprinkle on top. Serve and enjoy.

Nutrition:

Calories 169

Fat 16.1

Fiber 2.8

Carbs 4.4

Protein 4

39. Turkey Breast With Maple Mustard Glaze

Preparation time: 10 minutes

Cooking time: 30 minutes

Servings: 4-6

Ingredients:

- 1 tablespoon of ghee

- 2 tablespoons Dijon mustard

- 1/4 cup maple syrup

- 1/2 teaspoon black pepper, freshly ground

- 1 teaspoon salt

- 1/2 teaspoon smoked paprika

- 1/2 teaspoon dried sage

- 1 teaspoon dried thyme

- 5-pound whole turkey breast

- 2 teaspoons olive oil

Directions

1. To begin with, preheat your Air fryer to 350F.

2. Then brush olive oil over the turkey breast to coat it.

3. Combine pepper, salt, paprika, sage and thyme and then rub the seasonings on the turkey breast.

4. Place the seasoned turkey breast to the basket of Air fryer and cook for 25 minutes on the pre-heated oven.

5. Flip over the breast and then fry the other side for about 12 minutes. Check whether the internal temperature has reached 165F, which means the meat is fully cooked.

6. Meanwhile, mix together ghee, mustard and maple syrup in a small saucepan. After the turkey breast is cooked, turn it to an upright position and brush graze all over.

7. Then air fry for another 5 minutes until the skin is brown and crispy. Allow the turkey breast to cool when loosely covered with foil for about 5-10 minutes then slice and serve.

Nutrition:

Calories 119

Fat 8.1

Fiber 1.4

Carbs 11.1

Protein 3

40. Chicken Soup

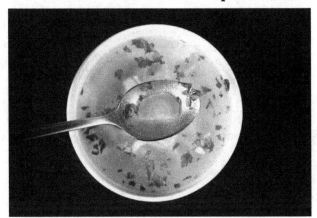

Preparation time: 10 minutes

Cooking time: 1 hour 30 minutes

Servings: 4-6

Ingredients:

- 1700ml water

- 4 chicken drum sticks

- 2 celery stalks

- 1-2 carrots

- 1 onion

- 1 tablespoon salt

- Pinch pepper

Directions:

1. Pre-heat a saucepan over medium heat, add water.

2. Wash the vegetables and dry them with paper towels.

3. Chop the ends of carrots and celery stalks. Skin the onion.

4. Put all the ingredients into the saucepan, cover with the lid and simmer for 90 minutes stirring from time to time.

5. As the soup is ready, separate the chicken meat from bones and add to the soup.

6. Pour the soup in the bowls.

Nutrition:

Calories 76

Fat 4.3

Fiber 0.3

Carbs 2.2

Protein 7.4

41. Fish Cakes

Preparation time: 15 minutes

Cooking time: 10 minutes

Servings: 4

Ingredients:

For The Fish Cakes

- 2 (6-ounce) fillets white fish

- 2 tablespoons almond flour

- 1 large shallot, minced

- 1/4 cup Homemade Mayo (here)

- Zest of 1 lemon

- Juice of 1/2 lemon

- 1/4 cup minced fresh parsley

- 2 tablespoons Dijon mustard

- 1 large egg, slightly beaten

- 1 teaspoon ground paprika

- Salt

- Freshly ground black pepper

- 2 tablespoons extra-virgin olive oil

For The Chili Sauce

- 2 tablespoons hot chili oil

- 1/4 cup apple cider vinegar

- 1/4 cup olive oil

To Serve

- 1/2 cup mizuna (or other lettuce)

- 1/2 cup arugula

- 1 carrot, julienned

- 1 small red Chile, sliced

Directions:

1. Chop the fish into a fine mince, and place in a large bowl.

2. Add the almond flour, shallot, Homemade Mayo, lemon zest and juice, parsley, mustard, egg, paprika, salt, and pepper, and mix well. Shape the mixture into four large cakes or eight smaller ones (smaller will be easier to turn over when cooking).

3. Set a large nonstick sauté pan over medium-high heat, heat the olive oil. Add the fish cakes, and allow them to brown, 4 to 5 minutes. Gently flip each one, reshaping as needed, and brown the other side, 4 to 5 minutes more.

For the chili sauce, combine all ingredients in a small bowl.

4. To serve, layer greens, carrot, and chills on serving plates, and top with fish cakes and chili sauce as desired.

Nutrition

Calories: 230

Fat: 10g

Carbs: 12g

Protein: 13g

Fiber: 4g

Sugar: 0g

42. Citrus-Baked Fish

Preparation time: 10 minutes

Cooking time: 15 minutes

Servings: 4

Ingredients:

- Ingredients: 2 lemons, sliced, divided

- 3 limes, sliced, divided

- 4 to 6 (6-ounce) fillets white fish (such as cod)

- Salt

- Freshly ground black pepper

- 1 tablespoon chopped fresh dill

- 1 tablespoon chopped fresh parsley

Directions:

1. Preheat the oven to 400F.

2. Set an 8-by-12-inch baking dish, layer half of the sliced lemons and limes to cover the bottom of the pan. Set with the fish fillets, and season with salt and pepper.

3. Layer the remaining lemon and lime slices on top, and bake for 10 to 15 minutes.

4. Remove from the oven, and serve the fish topped with the dill and parsley.

Nutrition

Calories: 170

Fat: 10g

Carbs: 2g

Protein: 22g

Fiber: 0g

Sugar: 0g

43. Poached Fish With Vegetables

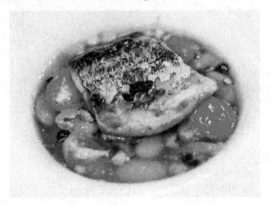

Preparation time: 10 minutes

Cooking time: 15 minutes

Servings: 2

Ingredients:

- 2 tablespoons grass-fed butter

- 2 (6-ounce) pieces white fish (such as cod or halibut)

- 1/2 cup diced onion

- 1/4 cup diced carrot

- 1/4 cup diced celery

- 2 or 3 fresh thyme sprigs, plus an extra pinch for garnish

- 1 large rosemary sprig, plus an extra pinch for garnish

- 2 or 3 fresh sage leaves (or pinch dried)

- 1 cup vegetable broth

- Salt

- Freshly ground black pepper

Directions:

1. In a skillet over medium-high heat, melt the butter. Quickly sear the fish, about 1 minute on each side. Detach it from the pan, and add the onion, carrot, celery, thyme, rosemary, and sage to the pan. Stir and sauté for 5 minutes.

2. Pour the vegetable broth into the skillet, and bring to a simmer. Return the fish to the skillet, and slowly poach until cooked throughout, 5 to 7 minutes.

3. Flavor with salt and pepper, and serve garnished with more fresh herbs.

Nutrition:

Calories: 32

Fat: 5

Fiber: 2

Carbs: 11

Protein: 4

44. Roasted Nut Mix

Preparation time: 10 minutes

Cooking time: 10 minutes

Servings: 6

Ingredients:

- 3 pecans, chopped

- 1/2 cup almonds, chopped

- 1/4 cup walnuts, chopped

- 1/2 cup hazelnuts, chopped

- 1 tablespoon avocado oil

- 1 teaspoon salt

Directions:

1. Heat up the avocado oil in the skillet and add chopped pecans, almonds, walnuts, and hazelnuts.

2. Add salt and mix up the mixture.

3. Roast it for 10 minutes on the medium heat. Stir the nut mix frequently.

Nutrition:

Calories 169

Fat 16.1

Fiber 2.8

Carbs 4.4

Protein 4.6

45. Raspberry And Apple Fruit Leather

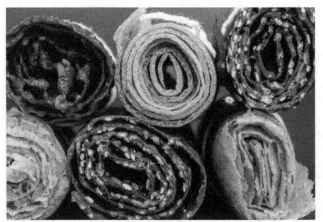

Preparation time: 10 minutes

Cooking time: 45 minutes

Servings: 6

Ingredients:

- 1 cup raspberries

- 1/2 cup apple, chopped

Directions:

1. Preheat the oven to 345F.

2. Line the baking tray with baking paper.

3. After this, put the raspberries and apples in the blender and blend until you get a smooth mixture.

4. Pour it in the baking tray and flatten well.

5. Bake the mixture for 45 minutes or until it is dry.

6. Then cut it into strips and roll into rolls.

Nutrition

Calories 20

Fat 0.2

Fiber 1.8

Carbs 5

Protein 0.3

46. Baked Apple With Hazelnuts

Preparation time: 15 minutes

Cooking time: 20 minutes

Servings: 8

Ingredients:

- 4 Granny Smith apples

- 4 teaspoons almond butter

- 2 tablespoons raw honey

- 2 oz. hazelnuts, chopped

Directions:

1. Cut the apples into halves and remove seeds.

2. Then make the medium size holes in the apple halves and fill them with almond butter, raw honey, and hazelnuts.

3. Place the apples in the tray and bake for 20 minutes at 350F.

Nutrition:

Calories 167

Fat 9

Fiber 4.2

Carbs 22.4

Protein 3.1

47. Banana Mini Muffins

Preparation time: 10 minutes

Cooking time: 10 minutes

Servings: 2

Ingredients:

- 2 eggs, beaten

- 1 banana, peeled

- 1/4 teaspoon ground cinnamon

Directions:

1. Mash the banana with the help of the fork until it is smooth.

2. Then add ground cinnamon and eggs. Stir the mixture well.

3. Pour the egg-banana mixture in the non-sticky muffin molds and bake at 365F for 10 minutes.

Nutrition:

Calories 116

Fat 4.6

Fiber 1.7

Carbs 14.1

Protein 6.2

48. Nuts And Raisins Apple Rings

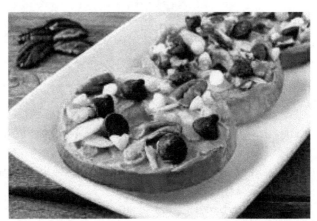

Preparation time: 15 minutes

Cooking time: 0 minutes

Servings: 5

Ingredients:

- 2 big apples

- 2 tablespoons raisins

- 2 tablespoons hazelnuts, chopped

- 1 tablespoon almond butter

Directions:

1. Core the apples and slice them.

2. Then mix up together raisins and hazelnuts.

3. Spread the apple slices with almond butter and sprinkle with hazelnut mixture.

Nutrition:

Calories 89

Fat 3.1

Fiber 2.8

Carbs 16.1

Protein 1.3

49. Chocolate Energy Balls

Preparation time: 15 minutes

Cooking time: 0 minutes

Servings: 5

Ingredients:

- 4 dates, chopped

- 3 oz. cashew, chopped

- 1 tablespoon cocoa powder

Directions:

1. Set the dates in the blender and blend until you get a smooth mixture.

2. Then add cashew and cocoa powder.

3. Blend mixture for 30 seconds more.

4. Then remove it from the blender and make 5 energy balls with the help of the fingertips.

Nutrition:

Calories 119

Fat 8.1

Fiber 1.4

Carbs 11.1

Protein 3

50. Turkey Sticks

Preparation time: 15 minutes

Cooking time: 10 minutes

Servings: 4

Ingredients:

- 6 oz. turkey breast, skinless, boneless

- 1 teaspoon tomato paste

- 1/2 teaspoon ground turmeric

- 1 tablespoon olive oil

- 1/2 teaspoon lemon juice

Directions:

1. Cut the turkey breast on medium-size sticks (strips).

2. Then mix up together tomato paste and olive oil.

3. Add lemon juice and ground turmeric.

4. After this, mix up turkey sticks and oil mixture.

5. Preheat the skillet until it is hot.

6. Put the turkey sticks in the skillet in one layer and roast them for 5 minutes from each side or until they turkey sticks are a little bit crunchy.

Nutrition:

Calories 76

Fat 4.3

Fiber 0.3

Carbs 2.2

Protein 7.4

51. Veggie Sticks

Preparation time: 10 minutes

Cooking time: 0 minutes

Servings: 4

Ingredients:

- 1 red sweet pepper

- 2 celery stalks

- 1 carrot, peeled

- 1 teaspoon coconut cream

- 1/4 teaspoon tahini paste

Directions:

1. Cut the sweet pepper, celery stalk, and carrot into the sticks.

2. Then put them in the plate side-by-side and sprinkle with coconut cream and tahini paste.

Nutrition:

Calories 22

Fat 0.6

Fiber 1

Carbs 4.1

Protein 0.6

CONCLUSION

The Paleo diet is a lifestyle answer that has been steadily gaining popularity these days. Many people are finding this diet very beneficial to their health. It is a natural diet that focuses on whole, unprocessed foods.

With the Paleo diet, you can lose weight and feel healthier. The Paleo diet is low in sugar. It is free of grains, dairy products, legumes, refined carbohydrates, and processed foods. This means that you get to eat natural foods rich in vitamins, minerals, antioxidants, and fiber.

The Paleo diet helps in the prevention of various diseases. Some of the Paleo diet benefits include an improved immune system and a reduction of chances of developing certain kinds of cancer and heart disease. This paleo diet is a manner of eating that became popular in the early 2000s. It's a lifestyle that hunter-gatherers have practiced for millions of years before the advent of agriculture. One of the main ideas behind this is that we are evolved to eat foods that are in season at the time. It's a way to ensure we get nutrients from our food. A straightforward way to implement this way of eating is to find whole, fresh foods that are in season at the time.